I0782951

Chair Yoga for Women over 50

A Safe and Supportive 28-Day Guide to Weight Loss, Balance and Well-being in the Comfort of Your Own Chair

Christoph Hermann

All rights reserved. No part of this book may be reproduced, stored in a retrieval system, or transmitted in any form or by any means, electronic, mechanical, photocopying, recording, or otherwise, without the prior written permission of the author, except for brief quotations embodied in critical reviews and certain other noncommercial uses permitted by copyright law.

Permission is granted to use brief excerpts in reviews or articles, provided proper credit is given to the author and the book.

The scanning, uploading, and distribution of this book via the internet or any other means without the permission of the author is illegal and punishable by law. Please purchase only authorized editions and support the author's work.

Copyright © Christoph Hermann, 2024

Disclaimer

The information and exercises presented in this book are for educational purposes only and are not intended to replace medical advice or treatment. Chair yoga is a gentle and modified form of yoga, but it is still important to consult with a healthcare professional before starting any new exercise program, especially if you have any underlying medical conditions or concerns.

The author and publisher of this book are not responsible for any injuries or damages that may result from practicing the exercises contained within. It is important to listen to your body and modify or stop practicing if you experience any discomfort or pain.

Additionally, the information and exercises presented in this book are not intended to be used as a substitute for professional medical treatment or therapy. If you are experiencing any physical or mental health issues, please seek help from a qualified healthcare professional.

By reading and using the information and exercises presented in this book, you acknowledge that you have read and understood this disclaimer and release the author and publisher from any liability.

Please practice yoga safely and responsibly!

Introduction

Understanding Chair Yoga

Chair Yoga is a modified version of traditional yoga that is practiced while seated or using a chair for support. This adaptation makes it an excellent option for individuals who face mobility issues or limitations, are recovering from injuries or surgery, or suffer from chronic pain or conditions like arthritis. Additionally, those who require a gentle and low-impact exercise routine, or are new to yoga and seeking a beginner-friendly practice, can greatly benefit from Chair Yoga.

The practice of Chair Yoga is designed to be accessible and inclusive, allowing individuals to engage in a yoga practice that may have previously been challenging or impossible due to physical limitations. By utilizing a chair for support and balance, participants can confidently explore various yoga poses and movements, knowing that they have a stable foundation to rely on.

The gentle stretches and movements incorporated into Chair Yoga are tailored to accommodate physical limitations, ensuring that participants can safely engage in the practice without exacerbating existing conditions or injuries. Deep breathing and relaxation techniques are also integral components of Chair Yoga, promoting relaxation and calmness, and helping to reduce stress and anxiety.

The emphasis on proper alignment and posture in Chair Yoga ensures that participants can maintain proper body positioning, even when using a chair for support. This focus on alignment and posture helps to build strength, improve flexibility, and enhance overall physical fitness, making Chair Yoga an excellent option for those seeking a low-impact yet effective exercise routine.

By engaging in Chair Yoga, individuals can experience a range of benefits that enhance their overall physical and mental well-being. Improved flexibility and range of motion, reduced stress and anxiety, enhanced balance and coordination, strengthened muscles, and increased energy levels are just a few of the advantages of incorporating Chair Yoga into one's routine. Additionally, Chair Yoga provides an opportunity for social interaction and community building, as participants can engage in group classes and workshops, sharing their experiences and supporting one another in their yoga journeys.

Overall, Chair Yoga offers a gentle yet powerful practice that can be adapted to suit individual needs and abilities, making it an accessible and inclusive form of yoga for all. Whether seeking a gentle exercise routine, a stress-reducing practice, or a community of like-minded individuals, Chair Yoga provides a welcoming and supportive environment for individuals to explore the benefits of yoga.

The Benefits of Chair Yoga

1. Gentle Empowerment:

Chair Yoga offers a sense of empowerment and control, allowing individuals to take charge of their physical and mental well-being in a gentle and accessible way.

2. Pain Relief and Management:

Chair Yoga provides a safe and effective way to manage chronic pain, arthritis, and other conditions, helping to reduce discomfort and improve overall quality of life.

3. Improved Flexibility and Mobility:

By incorporating gentle stretches and movements, Chair Yoga helps to increase flexibility, range of motion, and mobility, making daily activities easier and more manageable.

4. Reduced Stress and Anxiety:

The deep breathing and relaxation techniques integrated into Chair Yoga help to calm the mind and body, reducing stress and anxiety and promoting a sense of calm and well-being.

5. **Enhanced Balance and Coordination:**

Chair Yoga improves balance, coordination, and overall physical stability, reducing the risk of falls and injuries.

6. **Increased Strength and Endurance:**

By engaging in Chair Yoga, individuals can build strength, endurance, and overall physical fitness, improving their ability to perform daily tasks and activities.

7. **Improved Posture and Alignment:**

The emphasis on proper alignment and posture in Chair Yoga helps to improve overall physical alignment, reducing the risk of injury and improving overall physical fitness.

8. Social Connection and Community:

Chair Yoga provides an opportunity for social interaction and community building, helping to combat loneliness and isolation.

9. Mind-Body Connection:

Chair Yoga fosters a deeper mind-body connection, promoting greater body awareness, self-awareness, and overall well-being.

10. Accessible and Inclusive:

Chair Yoga is an accessible and inclusive practice, accommodating physical limitations and abilities, making it an excellent option for individuals of all ages and fitness levels.

11.   Improved Sleep:

Regular Chair Yoga practice can lead to improved sleep quality, duration, and overall sleep hygiene.

12.   Boosted Energy and Vitality:

Chair Yoga helps to increase energy levels, reduce fatigue, and promote overall physical and mental vitality.

The Benefits of Chair Yoga for Elderly Women

As women age, they face unique physical and emotional challenges that can impact their overall health and well-being. Chair Yoga offers a gentle, accessible, and empowering practice that addresses these challenges, promoting healthy aging and enhancing quality of life. These are the benefits of Chair Yoga for elderly women:

1. Osteoporosis Prevention:

Chair Yoga helps maintain bone density, reducing the risk of osteoporosis and fractures.

2. Menopause Symptom Relief:

Chair Yoga alleviates menopause symptoms like hot flashes, mood swings, and sleep disturbances.

3. Improved Balance and Fall Prevention:

Chair Yoga enhances balance, coordination, and physical stability, reducing the risk of falls.

4. Arthritis Management:

Chair Yoga gently mobilizes joints, reducing stiffness and pain, and improving mobility.

5. Heart Health:

Chair Yoga lowers blood pressure, improves circulation, and reduces the risk of heart disease.

6. Cognitive Function and Memory:

Chair Yoga improves focus, concentration, and memory, reducing the risk of cognitive decline.

7. Emotional Well-being:

Chair Yoga promotes relaxation, reduces stress and anxiety, and enhances overall mental health.

8. Social Connection:

Chair Yoga classes provide opportunities for social interaction, combating loneliness and isolation.

9. Improved Sleep:

Regular Chair Yoga practice leads to better sleep quality, duration, and overall sleep hygiene.

10. Increased Energy and Vitality:

Chair Yoga boosts energy levels, reducing fatigue and promoting overall physical and mental vitality.

11. Self-Esteem and Empowerment:

Chair Yoga fosters a sense of accomplishment, self-esteem, and empowerment, promoting healthy aging and well-being.

12. Accessibility and Inclusivity:

Chair Yoga accommodates physical limitations, making it an excellent option for elderly women with mobility issues or chronic conditions.

How to Use This Book

Welcome to Chair Yoga for Women over 50! This book is designed to be a comprehensive guide for practicing Chair Yoga, tailored specifically to the needs and abilities of elderly women. Here's how to use this book to get the most out of your Chair Yoga practice:

1. **Start slow:** Begin with short practices (10-15 minutes) and gradually increase as you become more comfortable with the poses and breathing techniques.

2. **Listen to your body:** Honor your physical limitations and take regular breaks. If you experience discomfort or pain, stop and modify the pose or rest.

3. **Focus on breathing:** Deep, conscious breathing is essential in Chair Yoga. Pay attention to your breath, and use it to guide your movements and relaxation.

4. **Use a chair for support:** The chair is your anchor and support. Use it to maintain balance, stability, and comfort throughout the practices.

5. **Practice regularly:** Aim to practice Chair Yoga at least 2-3 times a week, ideally at the same time each day to establish a routine.

6. **Explore and modify:** Don't be afraid to explore different poses and modify them to suit your needs. This book offers variations and adaptations to accommodate physical limitations.

7. **Connect with your inner self:** Chair Yoga is not just physical; it's also

a mental and emotional practice. Take time to connect with your inner self, and cultivate mindfulness and self-awareness.

8. **Seek guidance:** If you're new to Chair Yoga or have concerns, consider working with a qualified instructor or healthcare professional to guide you.

9. **Make it a ritual:** Create a peaceful and calming environment for your Chair Yoga practice, and make it a special time for self-care and self-love.

10. **Enjoy the journey:** Chair Yoga is a journey, not a destination. Embrace the process, and celebrate small victories along the way.

Exploring Chair Yoga

The Origins and Evolution of Chair Yoga

Chair Yoga, a gentle and accessible form of yoga, has its roots in the early 1980s. **Lakshmi Voelker-Binder**, a pioneering yoga instructor, created this innovative practice in response to a student's need for a more adaptable and inclusive approach to traditional yoga. This student, struggling with arthritis, required a modified practice that could accommodate physical limitations while still delivering the benefits of yoga.

Voelker-Binder's vision was to make yoga accessible to everyone, regardless of age, ability, or physical condition. She drew upon her extensive knowledge of yoga and her experience working with students with varying needs to develop a unique and revolutionary approach. By incorporating a chair for support and stability, she created a practice that could be done while seated or standing, making it an ideal option for those who may have found traditional yoga challenging or impossible.

The chair became a symbol of empowerment, allowing individuals to take control of their physical and mental well-being. Voelker-Binder's approach emphasized gentle movements, deep breathing, and meditation, creating a holistic practice that nurtured the body, mind, and spirit.

Over the years, Chair Yoga has evolved and grown in popularity, becoming a staple in yoga studios, senior centers, and healthcare facilities worldwide. Its gentle and adaptable nature has made it an attractive option for individuals with physical limitations, chronic conditions, or those seeking a low-impact, stress-reducing practice.

As Chair Yoga continued to spread, it drew attention from healthcare professionals, who recognized its potential as a therapeutic tool. Studies began to emerge, highlighting its benefits for seniors, individuals with chronic pain, and those recovering from injuries or surgery.

Today, Chair Yoga continues to inspire and empower individuals of all ages and abilities, offering a holistic approach to mind-body wellness that is both nourishing and transformative. Its evolution is a testament to the power of innovation and the human spirit, demonstrating that yoga can be adapted and made accessible to everyone, regardless of physical limitations or mobility.

Chair Yoga has become a beacon of hope for those who thought yoga was beyond their reach. It has created a sense of community and belonging among its practitioners, who share a common goal of cultivating physical, mental, and emotional well-being.

As we look to the future, Chair Yoga is poised to continue its growth and evolution, reaching even more individuals and communities worldwide. Its impact will be felt for generations to come, as it leaves a lasting legacy of empowerment, inclusivity, and wellness for all.

The Principles and Philosophy of Chair Yoga

Chair Yoga is rooted in the timeless wisdom of traditional yoga, adapted to meet the needs of modern individuals. Its principles and philosophy are guided by the following core values:

1. **Inclusivity:** Chair Yoga is for every body, regardless of age, ability, or physical condition.

2. **Accessibility:** Modifications and adaptations make yoga accessible to all.

3. **Gentle Empowerment:** Encouraging self-care, self-awareness, and self-compassion.

4. **Breath-Centered:** Deep breathing and conscious awareness are the foundation of the practice.

5. Mind-Body Connection: Integrating physical postures, breathing techniques, and meditation for holistic well-being.

6. Non-Competitive: Focus on individual growth, not comparison or competition.

7. Self-Care: Prioritizing one's own well-being and nurturing inner peace.

8. Awareness and Acceptance: Honoring the present moment and embracing limitations.

9. Empowerment through Education: Teaching individuals to take ownership of their health and wellness.

10. **Compassion and Kindness:** Cultivating a supportive and inclusive community.

Safety Considerations for Women in Chair Yoga

1. **Listen to your body:** Honor your physical limitations and take regular breaks.

2. **Modify or avoid:** Certain poses may need modification or avoidance due to physical limitations or health conditions.

3. **Breathing and pacing:** Focus on deep breathing and pace yourself to avoid fatigue.

4. **Proper alignment:** Maintain proper alignment to avoid discomfort or injury.

5. **Support and stability:** Use the chair for support and stability when needed.

6. **Hydration and nutrition:** Stay hydrated and energized with nutritious snacks.

7. **Comfortable clothing:** Wear comfortable, breathable clothing.

8. **Personal space and boundaries:** Respect your personal space and boundaries.

9. **Informed instructor:** Practice with an instructor knowledgeable about women's health and safety considerations.

10. **Self-care and awareness:**
Prioritize self-care and awareness of your physical and emotional well-being.

Additionally, women should be mindful of specific health considerations, such as:

- Menstruation and menstruation-related discomfort
- Pregnancy and postpartum recovery
- Menopause and hormonal changes
- Breast health and sensitivity
- Pelvic floor health and stability

By prioritizing safety and awareness, women can enjoy the benefits of Chair Yoga while nurturing their physical, emotional, and mental well-being.

Getting Started with Chair Yoga

Setting Up Your Practice Space

1. **Dedicate a quiet space:** Designate a quiet, peaceful area for your practice, free from distractions.

2. **Comfortable seating:** Choose a sturdy, comfortable chair with good back support.

3. **Non-slip flooring:** Ensure the floor is non-slip and clear of obstacles.

4. **Soothing colors:** Surround yourself with calming colors, such as beige, blue, or green.

5. **Natural light:** Position yourself near a natural light source, if possible.

6. **Calm scents:** Use essential oils or scented candles with calming fragrances like lavender or vanilla.

7. **Minimal clutter:** Keep the space clutter-free and organized.

8. **Inspiring decor:** Add calming elements like plants, nature-inspired artwork, or a meditation bell.

9. **Temperature control:** Maintain a comfortable temperature between 68-72°F (20-22°C).

10. **Technology:** Consider using a timer, calming music, or guided meditation apps to enhance your practice.

Essential Equipment for Chair Yoga

1. **Sturdy Chair:** A comfortable, stable chair with good back support.

2. **Yoga Mat:** A non-slip, eco-friendly mat for grip and hygiene.

3. **Blocks and Straps:** For modifying poses and maintaining proper alignment.

4. **Blanket or Towel:** For comfort, grip, and sweat absorption.

5. **Bolster or Pillow:** For support and relaxation in seated and reclined poses.

6. **Timer:** To keep track of practice time and intervals.

7. **Calming Aids:** Soothing music, essential oils, or guided meditation apps.

8. **Water Bottle:** To stay hydrated during practice.

9. **Comfortable Clothing:** Loose, breathable clothing for ease of movement.

10. **Optional Props:** Weights, resistance bands, or a meditation bench for added variety and support.

Remember, the most essential equipment is your own body and breath. These tools simply enhance and support your Chair Yoga practice.

Comfortable Attire and Accessories for Chair Yoga

Attire:

- Loose, breathable clothing (natural fibers like cotton, bamboo, or linen)
- Comfortable pants or leggings
- Soft, supportive tops (t-shirts, tank tops, or blouses)
- Layers for temperature control (optional)

Accessories:

- Yoga socks or grip socks for traction
- Comfortable, supportive shoes (optional)
- Soft, breathable scarf or wrap (for warmth or style)
- Hair tie or clip (to keep hair out of face)
- Minimal jewelry (avoiding distractions or discomfort)

Chair Yoga Poses for Strength and Flexibility

Gentle Warm-Up Movements for Chair Yoga

Neck Stretch:

1. Sit comfortably with your back straight and feet planted firmly on the ground.
2. Slowly tilt your head to the right, bringing your ear towards your right shoulder.
3. Keep your chin straight and your head level.
4. Hold the stretch for 15-30 seconds, feeling the gentle stretch in your neck and shoulder.
5. Release and repeat on the left side.

Tips:

- Keep your shoulders relaxed and down.
- Avoid forcing or bouncing beyond a comfortable stretch.
- Breathe deeply and naturally, feeling the stretch in your neck and shoulder.

Shoulder Rolls:

1. Sit comfortably with your back straight and feet planted firmly on the ground.
2. Relax your shoulders and let them drop down, feeling any tension or stress melt away.
3. Roll your shoulders forward and up towards your ears, then back and down, creating a circular motion.
4. Repeat several times, moving slowly and smoothly.

5. Focus on the sensation of relaxation spreading through your shoulders and upper back.

Tips:

- Keep your chest open and your spine long.
- Avoid scrunching your shoulders or tensing your neck.
- Breathe naturally, feeling the relaxation spread through your shoulders with each roll.

Chest Expansion:

1. Sit comfortably with your back straight and feet planted firmly on the ground.
2. Place your hands on your thighs, just above your knees.

3. Take a deep breath in, feeling your chest expand and your shoulders relax.
4. As you inhale, press your hands into your thighs and gently arch your chest forward.
5. Hold the expansion for a moment, feeling the opening in your chest and shoulders.
6. Exhale slowly, releasing any tension or constriction.

Tips:

- Keep your shoulders down and relaxed.
- Avoid forcing or straining; focus on gentle expansion.
- Breathe naturally, feeling the opening in your chest with each breath.

Arm Circles:

1. Sit comfortably with your back straight and feet planted firmly on the ground.
2. Hold your arms straight out to the sides, parallel to the ground.
3. Make small circles with your hands for 5-10 repetitions.
4. Gradually increase the size of the circles as you continue.
5. Switch directions and repeat.

Tips:

- Keep your shoulders relaxed and down.
- Avoid tensing your arms or shoulders; focus on smooth, flowing circles.
- Breathe naturally, feeling the relaxation spread through your arms and shoulders.

Wrist Extensions:

1. Sit comfortably with your back straight and feet planted firmly on the ground.
2. Hold your arm straight out in front of you, palm down.
3. Slowly tilt your wrist up, keeping your arm still, and then lower it back down.
4. Repeat for 5-10 repetitions.
5. Switch arms and repeat.

Tips:

- Keep your arm straight and relaxed.
- Avoid bending your elbow or tensing your shoulder.
- Focus on the gentle movement of your wrist, feeling the stretch and relaxation.

Seated Twist:

1. Sit comfortably with your back straight and feet planted firmly on the ground.
2. Place your right hand on the outside of your left knee.
3. Gently twist your torso to the left, keeping your feet and hips facing forward.
4. Hold for a few breaths, feeling the stretch in your spine and torso.
5. Release and repeat on the other side by placing your left hand on the outside of your right knee.

Tips:

- Keep your spine long and your shoulders relaxed.
- Avoid forcing or bouncing; gentle twisting motion.

- Breathe naturally, feeling the stretch and relaxation spread through your torso.

Hip Openers:

1. Sit comfortably with your back straight and feet planted firmly on the ground.
2. Slowly slide your right foot away from your left foot, keeping your knees straight.
3. Hold the stretch for 15-30 seconds, feeling the opening in your hip and groin area.
4. Release and repeat on the left side.

Tips:

- Keep your back straight and your core engaged.

- Avoid bouncing or forcing beyond a comfortable stretch.
- Breathe deeply, feeling the opening and relaxation in your hips and lower back.

Note: If you experience any discomfort or pain, stop the stretch immediately and consult with a healthcare professional.

Ankle Rotations:

1. Sit comfortably with your back straight and feet planted firmly on the ground.
2. Lift your right foot off the ground, keeping your knee straight.
3. Rotate your ankle in a circular motion, starting from small circles and gradually increasing in size.

4. Repeat for 5-10 repetitions.
5. Switch to your left foot and repeat.

Tips:

- Keep your knee straight and your foot relaxed.
- Avoid bouncing or forcing; focus on smooth, flowing circles.
- Breathe naturally, feeling the relaxation spread through your ankles and feet.

Toe Wiggles:

1. Sit comfortably with your back straight and feet planted firmly on the ground.
2. Wiggle your toes, spreading them apart as far as you can.
3. Then, bring them back together, curling them under.

4. Repeat for 5-10 repetitions.
5. Focus on the movement of each toe, feeling the flexibility and relaxation in your feet.

Tips:

- Keep your feet flat on the ground.
- Avoid tensing your feet or ankles; focus on gentle, playful movements.
- Breathe naturally, feeling the relaxation spread through your toes and feet.

Deep Breathing:

- Take slow, deep breaths in through your nose and out through your mouth, focusing on the sensation of the breath.

These gentle warm-up movements prepare your body for Chair Yoga, increasing blood flow and flexibility while reducing stiffness and tension.

Seated Stretches for Supple Joints:

1. Seated Neck Stretch:

Slowly tilt your head to the side, bringing your ear towards your shoulder. Hold, then release. Repeat on the other side.

2. Seated Shoulder Rolls:

Roll your shoulders forward and backward in a circular motion. Repeat several times.

3. Seated Chest Expansion:

Place your hands on your thighs and take a deep breath in, expanding your chest. Exhale, relaxing your shoulders.

4. Seated Arm Circles:

Hold your arms straight out to the sides and make small circles with your hands. Gradually increase the size of the circles.

5. Seated Side Stretch:

Slowly lean to one side, keeping your feet on the floor. Hold, then release. Repeat on the other side.

6. Seated Hip Flexor Stretch:

Slowly lift your right foot off the ground, keeping your knee straight. Hold, then release. Repeat on the left side.

7. Seated Ankle Rotations:

Lift your right foot off the ground and rotate your ankle in a circular motion. Repeat on the left side.

8. Seated Toe Wiggles:

Wiggle your toes, spreading them apart and curling them under.

Building Strength in Key Muscles:

Chair Squats:

1. Stand up and sit down in your chair without using your hands.
2. Keep your back straight, engage your core, and lower yourself into a seated position.
3. Push through your legs to return to standing.
4. Repeat for 10-15 reps.

Tips:

- Keep your weight in your heels, not your toes.
- Avoid using your hands or arms to push yourself up or down.
- Focus on slow, controlled movements.
- Take breaks as needed.

Modifications:

- If standing and sitting is too challenging, try standing and lowering yourself into a seated position, then using your hands to push yourself back up.

- If you need more support, try holding onto the armrests or using a walker for balance.

Chair Leg Lifts:

1. Sit comfortably in your chair with your feet flat on the floor.
2. Lift one leg off the floor, keeping your knee straight.
3. Hold for a few seconds (about 2-3 seconds).
4. Lower your leg back down to the starting position.
5. Repeat with the other leg.
6. Continue alternating legs for 10-15 reps on each leg.

Tips:

- Keep your back straight and engage your core.
- Avoid using momentum or jerking movements.
- Focus on slow, controlled lifts and lowers.
- Take breaks as needed.

Modifications:

- If lifting your leg straight out is too challenging, try bending your knee and lifting your leg up towards your chest.

- If you need more support, try holding onto the armrests or using a walker for balance.

Arm Raises:

1. Sit comfortably in your chair with your feet flat on the floor.
2. Hold your arms straight out to the sides, parallel to the ground.
3. Raise one arm up towards the ceiling, keeping it straight.
4. Hold for a few seconds (about 2-3 seconds).
5. Lower your arm back down to the starting position.
6. Repeat with the other arm.
7. Continue alternating arms for 10-15 reps on each arm.

Tips:

- Keep your shoulders relaxed and down.
- Avoid using momentum or jerking movements.
- Focus on slow, controlled raises and lowers.

- Take breaks as needed.

Modifications:

- If raising your arm straight up is too challenging, try bending your elbow and lifting your hand up towards your shoulder.

- If you need more support, try holding onto the armrests or using a light weight in each hand.

Shoulder Blade Squeezes:

1. Sit comfortably in your chair with your feet flat on the floor.
2. Sit up straight and squeeze your shoulder blades together.
3. Hold for a few seconds (about 2-3 seconds).

4. Release and repeat for 10-15 reps.

Tips:

- Keep your shoulders relaxed and down.
- Avoid tensing your neck or shoulders.
- Focus on squeezing your shoulder blades together.
- Take breaks as needed.

Modifications:

- If you find it difficult to squeeze your shoulder blades together, try placing your hands on your shoulders and gently squeezing your shoulders together.

- If you need more support, try using a resistance band or a small towel to help squeeze your shoulder blades together.

Toe Taps:

1. Sit comfortably in your chair with your feet flat on the floor.
2. Lift your feet off the ground and tap your toes on the floor in front of you.
3. Tap your toes in a rhythmic motion, alternating feet.
4. Continue for 10-15 reps on each foot.

Tips:

- Keep your knees straight and your feet flexed.
- Avoid using momentum or jerking movements.
- Focus on quick, light taps.
- Take breaks as needed.

Modifications:

- If tapping your toes is too challenging, try lifting your feet off the ground and

holding them for a few seconds before
lowering.

- If you need more support, try using a
resistance band or a small towel to
help lift your feet.

Seated Marching:

1. Sit comfortably in your chair with your
feet flat on the floor.
2. Lift your feet off the ground and
march in place, keeping your knees
straight.
3. Alternate legs in a marching motion,
as if walking in place.
4. Continue for 10-15 reps on each leg.

Tips:

- Keep your back straight and engage your core.
- Avoid using momentum or jerking movements.
- Focus on quick, light steps.
- Take breaks as needed.

Modifications:

- If marching is too challenging, try lifting your feet off the ground and holding them for a few seconds before lowering.

- If you need more support, try using a resistance band or a small towel to help lift your legs.

Seated Leg Press:

1. Sit comfortably in your chair with your feet flat on the floor.
2. Push your legs against the floor, as if pushing off with your feet.
3. Keep your knees straight and your feet flexed.
4. Hold for a few seconds (about 2-3 seconds).
5. Release and repeat for 10-15 reps.

Tips:

- Engage your core and keep your back straight.
- Avoid using momentum or jerking movements.
- Focus on slow, controlled presses.
- Take breaks as needed.

Modifications:

-   If pushing your legs against the floor is too challenging, try lifting your feet off the ground and holding them for a few seconds before lowering.

-   If you need more support, try using a resistance band or a small towel to help push your legs against the floor.

Chair Yoga for Balance and Stability

Enhancing Balance with Chair Support:

Single-Leg Stand:

1. Stand beside the chair with your feet hip-width apart.
2. Hold the chair with one hand for support.
3. Slowly lift one foot off the ground, keeping your knee straight.
4. Hold the single-leg stand for 10-15 seconds.
5. Lower your foot back down to the starting position.
6. Repeat on the other side.

Tips:

- Keep your back straight and engage
  your core.
- Avoid leaning forward or backward.
- Focus on your balance and stability.
- Take breaks as needed.

Modifications:

- If you're new to single-leg stands, start
  with shorter holds (5-7 seconds) and
  gradually increase the time as you
  build balance and strength.

- If you need more support, hold the
  chair with both hands or use a walker
  for additional stability.

Heel-To-Toe Walks:

1. Stand beside the chair with your feet together.
2. Hold the chair with one hand for support.
3. Take a small step forward with one foot, placing the heel of that foot directly in front of the toes of the other foot.
4. Bring the other foot forward, placing its heel directly in front of the toes of the first foot.
5. Continue walking in this manner, alternating feet and keeping your knees straight.
6. Walk for 5-10 steps, then turn around and walk back to the starting position.

Tips:

- Keep your back straight and engage your core.

- Avoid looking down at the floor; instead, focus on a point in front of you.
- Take small, slow steps and concentrate on your balance.
- Take breaks as needed.

Modifications:

- If you're new to heel-to-toe walks, start with shorter distances (3-5 steps) and gradually increase the length as you build balance and strength.

- If you need more support, hold the chair with both hands or use a walker for additional stability.

Side Steps:

1. Stand beside the chair with your feet together.
2. Hold the chair with one hand for support.
3. Take a small step to one side with one foot (about 6-8 inches).
4. Bring the other foot to meet the first foot, so your feet are together again.
5. Take a small step to the other side with the first foot.
6. Continue alternating sides for 10-15 reps.

Tips:

- Keep your back straight and engage your core.
- Avoid leaning forward or backward.
- Focus on slow, controlled steps.
- Take breaks as needed.

Modifications:

- If you're new to side steps, start with smaller steps (about 4-6 inches) and gradually increase the distance as you build balance and strength.

- If you need more support, hold the chair with both hands or use a walker for additional stability.

Standing Leg Lifts:

1. Stand beside the chair with your feet hip-width apart.
2. Hold the chair with one hand for support.
3. Slowly lift one leg off the ground, keeping it straight.
4. Hold the leg lift for a few seconds (about 2-3 seconds).
5. Lower your leg back down to the starting position.
6. Repeat on the other side.

Tips:

- Keep your back straight and engage your core.
- Avoid leaning forward or backward.
- Focus on slow, controlled lifts.
- Take breaks as needed.

Modifications:

- If you're new to standing leg lifts, start with smaller lifts (about 2-3 inches off the ground) and gradually increase the height as you build strength and balance.

- If you need more support, hold the chair with both hands or use a walker for additional stability.

Eyes Closed Standing:

1. Stand beside the chair with your feet hip-width apart.
2. Hold the chair with one hand for support.
3. Close your eyes and take a deep breath.
4. Stand with your eyes closed for 10-15 seconds.
5. Open your eyes and take a deep breath.
6. Repeat for 3-5 reps.

Tips:

- Keep your back straight and engage your core.
- Focus on your balance and stability.
- Take slow, deep breaths.
- Take breaks as needed.

Modifications:

- If you're new to eyes closed standing, start with shorter holds (5-7 seconds) and gradually increase the time as you build balance and strength.

- If you need more support, hold the chair with both hands or use a walker for additional stability.

Preventing Falls Through Practice

Preventing Falls Through Practice is a crucial aspect of maintaining balance and stability. These are some exercises and tips to help you practice and reduce the risk of falls:

1. **Standing Up and Sitting Down:** Practice standing up and sitting down

without using your hands. Start with a chair and gradually move to a couch or bench.

2. **Walking and Turning:** Practice walking and turning in different directions. Focus on keeping your body straight and taking small steps.

3. **Heel-To-Toe Walks:** Walk along a straight line, placing the heel of one foot directly in front of the toes of the other foot.

4. **Single-Leg Stands:** Stand on one leg, holding onto a chair or wall for support. Gradually increase the time as you build balance.

5. **Reaching and Bending:** Practice reaching for objects and bending to pick up items. Focus on keeping your body straight and using your legs to lift.

6. **Vision Exercises:** Practice changing your focus between near and far objects. This will help improve your depth perception and balance.

7. **Reaction Time:** Practice reacting quickly to unexpected situations, such as a sudden noise or a loss of balance.

8. **Balance Games:** Play games that challenge your balance, such as standing on one foot while brushing your teeth or holding a balance board.

9. **Practice in Different Environments:** Practice your balance exercises in different environments, such as on a soft surface or a hard floor.

10. **Get Enough Sleep and Exercise:** Getting enough sleep and

regular exercise can help improve your balance and reduce the risk of falls.

Strengthening the core for Stability

This is essential for improving stability and balance. These are some exercises to help strengthen your core:

1. **Plank:** Hold a plank position for 30-60 seconds, rest for 30 seconds, and repeat for 3-5 reps.

2. **Bridge:** Lie on your back with knees bent and feet flat on the floor. Lift your hips up towards the ceiling, squeezing your core muscles, and hold for 2-3 seconds. Repeat for 10-15 reps.

3. **Pelvic Tilt:** Lie on your back with knees bent and feet flat on the floor. Tilt your pelvis upwards and then back down again, repeating the motion for 10-15 reps.

4. **Leg Raises:** Lie on your back with arms extended overhead and legs straight. Lift your legs off the ground, keeping them straight, and hold for 2-3 seconds. Repeat for 10-15 reps.

5. **Russian twists:** Sit on the floor with knees bent and feet flat. Lean back slightly and lift your feet off the ground. Hold a weight or medicine ball and twist your torso from side to side, touching the weight to the ground beside you. Repeat for 10-15 reps.

6. **Bicycle crunches:** Lie on your back with hands behind your head and legs

lifted and bent at a 90-degree angle. Alternate bringing your knees towards your chest, as if pedaling a bicycle. Repeat for 10-15 reps.

7. **Pallof press:** Hold a resistance band or cable handle and stand with your feet shoulder-width apart. Press the handle away from your body, keeping your core muscles engaged, and hold for 2-3 seconds. Repeat for 10-15 reps.

Chair Yoga for Balance and Stability

Breathing Techniques for Relaxation

- **Diaphragmatic Breathing**

This is also known as **belly breathing**, this technique engages your diaphragm to breathe deeply into your lungs. Place one hand on your belly and the other on your chest. Inhale deeply through your nose, allowing your belly to rise while your chest remains still. Exhale slowly through your mouth, allowing your belly to fall.

- **4-7-8 Breathing**

This is also known as the **"Relaxation Breath"** or **"Complete Breath,"** is a simple yet powerful breathing exercise that can help calm your mind and body. Here's how to do it:

1. Find a comfortable and quiet place to sit or lie down.
2. Close your eyes and take a deep breath in through your nose for a count of 4.

3. Hold your breath for a count of 7.
4. Slowly exhale through your mouth for a count of 8.
5. Repeat the cycle for several rounds, ideally 3-5 minutes.

This technique works by:

- Slowing down your heart rate and promoting relaxation
- Reducing stress and anxiety by activating the parasympathetic nervous system
- Increasing oxygenation of the body and brain
- Helping to quiet the mind and promote a sense of calm

- **Box Breathing**

Box breathing, also known as **square breathing**, is a simple yet powerful breathing technique that can help calm your mind and body. Here's how to do it:

1. Find a comfortable and quiet place to sit or lie down.
2. Close your eyes and take a deep breath in for a count of 4, filling your lungs completely.
3. Hold your breath for a count of 4.
4. Slowly exhale for a count of 4, emptying your lungs completely.
5. Hold your breath again for a count of 4.
6. Repeat the cycle for several rounds, ideally 3-5 minutes.

This technique works by:

- Slowing down your heart rate and promoting relaxation
- Reducing stress and anxiety by activating the parasympathetic nervous system

- Increasing oxygenation of the body and brain
- Helping to quiet the mind and promote a sense of calm

The **"box"** shape comes from the equal lengths of the breaths:

- Inhale for 4 counts (top of the box)
- Hold for 4 counts (right side of the box)
- Exhale for 4 counts (bottom of the box)
- Hold for 4 counts (left side of the box)

- **Alternate Nostril Breathing (Nadi Shodhana)**

This is another yogic breathing technique that helps balance the breath, calm the mind, and prepare for meditation. Here's how to perform it:

1. Find a comfortable seated position with your back straight.
2. Place your right hand in front of your face, with your thumb and pinky finger forming a "V" shape.
3. Close your right nostril with your thumb and inhale through your left nostril.
4. Close your left nostril with your pinky finger and exhale through your right nostril.
5. Inhale through your right nostril, closing your left nostril with your pinky finger.
6. Exhale through your left nostril, closing your right nostril with your thumb.
7. Repeat for several rounds, ideally 3-5 minutes.

This technique helps:

- Balance the breath and calm the mind

- Prepare for meditation and relaxation
- Reduce stress and anxiety
- Improve respiratory function
- Balance the left and right hemispheres of the brain

- **Progressive Muscle Relaxation with Breathing**

Progressive Muscle Relaxation **(PMR)** with breathing is a powerful technique to reduce stress, anxiety, and muscle tension. Here's a step-by-step guide:

1. Find a comfortable and quiet place to lie down or sit comfortably.
2. Start with deep breathing: inhale for 4 counts, hold for 4 counts, and exhale for 4 counts. Repeat this cycle a few times.
3. Tense and then relax different muscle groups in your body, starting with:

- Toes and feet (tense for 5-7 seconds, release and feel the relaxation spread)
- Calves and ankles
- Thighs
- Hips and lower back
- Upper back and shoulders
- Arms and hands
- Neck and head

4. As you tense each muscle group, hold for 5-7 seconds and then release and feel the relaxation spread through your muscles.
5. Take deep breaths between each muscle group, focusing on the sensation of relaxation spreading through your body.
6. Repeat the cycle 2-3 times, taking breaks to breathe deeply and relax further.

Tips:

- Start with lighter tension and gradually increase as needed.
- Focus on the sensation of relaxation spreading through your muscles.
- Use a guided recording or a partner to help you stay focused.
- Practice regularly to reduce overall stress and anxiety.

- **Visualization with Breathing**

1. Find a quiet and comfortable place to sit or lie down.
2. Close your eyes and take a few deep breaths, focusing on the sensation of the breath moving in and out of your body.
3. Imagine yourself in a peaceful, relaxing environment (e.g., a beach, forest, or mountain meadow).
4. Visualize this place in as much detail as possible, using all your senses:

- See the vibrant colors and textures.
- Hear the soothing sounds (e.g., waves, birdsong, or wind).
- Smell the scents (e.g., salty air, flowers, or pine).
- Feel the sensations (e.g., warm sun, cool breeze, or soft grass).

5. As you breathe in, imagine fresh, calming air filling your lungs and spreading throughout your body.
6. As you breathe out, imagine any stress, anxiety, or tension leaving your body.
7. Continue visualizing and breathing deeply for several minutes, allowing yourself to fully relax and unwind.
8. When you're ready, slowly open your eyes, and take a moment to notice how you feel before getting up and going about your day.

Tips:

- Use a guided visualization recording to help you get started.
- Incorporate elements that evoke a sense of calm and relaxation, such as water, nature, or peaceful music.
- Practice regularly to enhance the effectiveness of this technique.
- Remember to breathe deeply and slowly, focusing on the sensation of the breath.

• **Equal Breathing (Sama Vritti)**

1. Find a comfortable seated or lying position.
2. Close your eyes and take a few deep breaths.
3. Inhale for a count of 4, filling your lungs completely.
4. Exhale for a count of 4, emptying your lungs completely.

5. Repeat this cycle, focusing on making your inhales and exhales equal in length.
6. Continue for several minutes, ideally 5-10.

Benefits:

- Calms the mind and body
- Reduces stress and anxiety
- Improves focus and concentration
- Enhances relaxation and sleep
- Balances the breath and nervous system

Tips:

- Start with shorter counts (e.g., 2-3) and gradually increase as you become more comfortable with the technique.
- Use a guided recording or a breathing app to help you stay focused.
- Practice regularly to experience the benefits.

- Remember to breathe naturally and smoothly, without forcing or controlling the breath too much.

- **Bellows Breath (Bhastrika Pranayama)**

1. Sit comfortably with your back straight.
2. Take a few deep breaths to relax.
3. Inhale and exhale rapidly through your nose, using your diaphragm to pump air in and out of your lungs.
4. Imagine a bellows expanding and contracting as you breathe.
5. Continue for 1-3 minutes, then take a few deep breaths and relax.

Benefits:

- Energizes and balances the body and mind

- Stimulates the respiratory and nervous systems
- Helps remove stale air and toxins from the lungs
- Improves oxygenation and circulation
- Enhances focus and concentration.

Tips:

- Start slowly and gradually increase the pace and duration.
- Use a guided recording or a breathing app to help you stay focused.
- Practice regularly to experience the benefits.
- Remember to breathe naturally and smoothly, without forcing or controlling the breath too much.

- **Sama Vritti (Equal Breathing)**

Benefits:

- Calms the mind and body
- Reduces stress and anxiety
- Improves focus and concentration
- Enhances relaxation and sleep
- Balances the breath and nervous system

How to practice:

1. Find a comfortable seated or lying position
2. Close your eyes and take a few deep breaths
3. Inhale for a count of 4, filling your lungs completely
4. Exhale for a count of 4, emptying your lungs completely
5. Repeat this cycle, focusing on making your inhales and exhales equal in length
6. Continue for several minutes, ideally 5-10

Tips:

- Start with shorter counts (e.g., 2-3) and gradually increase as you become more comfortable with the technique
- Use a guided recording or a breathing app to help you stay focused
- Practice regularly to experience the benefits
- Remember to breathe naturally and smoothly, without forcing or controlling the breath too much

- **Bhastrika Breathing (Bhastrika Pranayama)**

Benefits:

- Energizes and balances the body and mind
- Stimulates the respiratory and nervous systems

- Helps remove stale air and toxins from the lungs
- Improves oxygenation and circulation
- Enhances focus and concentration

How to practice:

1. Sit comfortably with your back straight
2. Take a few deep breaths to relax
3. Inhale and exhale rapidly through your nose, using your diaphragm to pump air in and out of your lungs
4. Imagine a bellows expanding and contracting as you breathe
5. Continue for 1-3 minutes, then take a few deep breaths and relax

Tips:

- Start slowly and gradually increase the pace and duration

- Use a guided recording or a breathing app to help you stay focused
- Practice regularly to experience the benefits
- Remember to breathe naturally and smoothly, without forcing or controlling the breath too much

Precautions:

- Avoid practicing Bhastrika Breathing if you have any respiratory issues or concerns

- If you experience dizziness or discomfort, stop and rest

Calming Poses for Body and Mind

- **Child's Pose (Balasana)**

1. Kneel on the mat with your knees wide apart.
2. Sit back onto your heels.
3. Stretch your arms out in front of you, lowering your forehead to the ground.
4. Take deep breaths, feeling the stretch in your back and the calmness in your mind.
5. Hold for 5-10 breaths, or as long as feels comfortable.
6. Slowly lift your forehead, then your arms, and finally your torso, returning to a seated position.

Tips:

- Keep your knees wide apart to allow for a comfortable stretch in your back.

- If your forehead doesn't reach the
  ground, you can use a block or a
  folded blanket to support your head.
- Take slow, deep breaths, focusing on
  the sensation of the breath moving in
  and out of your body.
- If you feel any discomfort or pain,
  come out of the pose immediately.

Benefits:

- Stretches the back, hips, and legs
- Calms the mind and promotes
  relaxation
- Can help reduce stress and anxiety
- Great for taking a break during a yoga
  practice or anytime you need a quick
  relaxation pose.

- **Cat-Cow   Pose
  (Marjaryasana-Bitilasana):**

Start on your hands and knees. Inhale, arching your back and lifting your tailbone (like a cat). Exhale, rounding your back and tucking your chin to your chest (like a cow). Repeat several times.

- **Downward-Facing Dog (Adho Mukha Svanasana):**

Start on your hands and knees. Walk your hands forward, lifting your hips up and back, straightening your arms and legs. Keep your head in a neutral position, breathing deeply.

- **Seated Forward Fold (Paschimottanasana):**

Sit on the ground with your legs extended in front of you. Inhale, lengthening your spine. Exhale, folding forward, reaching for your toes or shins. Hold for several breaths.

- **Pigeon Pose (Eka Pada Rajakapotasana):**

Start on your hands and knees. Bring one knee forward, placing your foot on the ground in front of the other knee. Lower your hips down, stretching the back leg. Switch sides.

- **Legs Up The Wall Pose (Viparita Karani):**

Lie on your back with your legs straight up against a wall. Relax your body, breathing deeply, and stay for several minutes.

- **Savasana (Corpse Pose):**

Lie on your back with your arms and legs relaxed. Close your eyes, focusing on your breath, and stay for several minutes.

- **Tree Pose (Vrksasana):**

Stand on one leg, with the other foot resting on the inner thigh. Engage your core, lift your arms overhead, and gaze forward. Switch legs.

- **Seated Twist (Bharadvajasana):**

Sit on the ground with your legs crossed. Twist your torso to one side, placing your hand on the outside of your knee. Look over your shoulder and hold for several breaths. Switch sides.

- **Sphinx Pose (Salamba Bhujangasana):**

Lie on your stomach with your forearms on the ground and lift your chest and head off the mat. Keep your shoulders down and away from your ears, breathing deeply.

Incorporating meditation into your practice

1. **Start small:** Begin with short meditation sessions (5-10 minutes) and gradually increase the duration as you become more comfortable with the practice.

2. **Find a quiet space:** Identify a quiet, comfortable spot where you can meditate without distractions.

3. **Focus on your breath:** Bring your attention to your breath, noticing the sensation of the air moving in and out of your body.

4. **When your mind wanders, gently bring it back:** Don't try to force your mind to stay focused, but rather gently bring it back to your breath when you notice it wandering.

5. **Be consistent:** Aim to meditate at the same time each day to make it a habit.

6. **Use guided meditations:** Listen to guided meditations to help you get started and stay focused.

7. **Be patient with yourself:** Remember that meditation is a practice, and it's okay if your mind wanders.

8. **Incorporate mindfulness into your daily activities:** Bring mindfulness into your daily routine by paying attention to your thoughts, emotions, and physical sensations.

9. **Experiment with different types of meditation:** Try various techniques, such as loving-kindness meditation, body scan meditation, or

transcendental meditation, to find what works best for you.

10. **Make it a ritual:** Create a peaceful pre-meditation routine, such as lighting a candle or sipping tea, to signal to your mind that it's time to meditate.

Chair Yoga for Women's Health Concerns

Alleviating Menopause Symptoms

1. **Hormone Replacement Therapy (HRT):**

Consult your healthcare provider about HRT options, which can help alleviate hot flashes, night sweats, and vaginal dryness.

2. **Phytoestrogens:**

Plant-based estrogens, found in foods like soy, flaxseeds, and fermented soy products, can help ease symptoms.

3. Herbal Remedies:

Black cohosh, dong quai, and valerian root may help with hot flashes, sleep disturbances, and mood swings.

4. Mind-Body Therapies:

Yoga, tai chi, and meditation can reduce stress, anxiety, and hot flashes.

5. Acupuncture:

This ancient practice may help balance hormones and alleviate symptoms.

6. Dietary Changes:

Eat a balanced diet rich in whole foods, fruits, vegetables, and omega-3 fatty acids to support overall health.

7. Stay Hydrated:

Drink plenty of water to help with vaginal dryness and overall health.

8. Exercise Regularly:

Engage in physical activities that bring you joy, like walking, swimming, or dancing, to help with mood and overall well-being.

9. Get Enough Sleep:

Prioritize restful sleep and aim for 7-8 hours per night.

10. Seek Support:

Connect with friends, family, or a therapist for emotional support and connection.

Managing Osteoporosis with Careful Movements

1. Gentle movements:

Avoid jerky or bouncy movements, which can put stress on fragile bones. Instead, focus on slow, controlled movements.

2. Strengthening poses:

Incorporate chair yoga poses that strengthen the muscles in your arms, legs, and core, such as chair squats, chair lunges, and chair leg lifts.

3. Balance and coordination:

Practice chair yoga poses that challenge your balance and coordination, such as single-leg stands and heel-to-toe walks.

4. Flexibility and stretching:

Gentle stretching can help improve flexibility and reduce stiffness. Focus on chair yoga poses that stretch your major muscle groups, such as chair forward bends and chair side stretches.

5. Breathing and relaxation:

Chair yoga can also help with deep breathing and relaxation techniques, which can reduce stress and promote overall well-being.

Some specific chair yoga poses for managing **osteoporosis** include:

- Chair mountain pose (strengthens core and legs)

- Chair tree pose (improves balance and coordination)
- Chair cat-cow pose (gently stretches spine and improves flexibility)
- Chair seated forward bend (stretches back, shoulders, and hips)
- Chair leg raises (strengthens legs and hips)

Improving Heart Health and Circulation

1. Gentle Cardiovascular Exercise:

Chair yoga can provide a gentle cardiovascular workout, helping to improve heart health and increase blood flow.

2. Improved Circulation:

Chair yoga poses can help improve circulation, which can increase oxygenation of the body and reduce inflammation.

3. Reduced Blood Pressure:

Regular chair yoga practice has been shown to help reduce blood pressure and improve overall cardiovascular health.

4. Increased Flexibility and Mobility:

Chair yoga can help improve flexibility and mobility, making it easier to move and perform daily activities.

5. Stress Reduction:

Chair yoga can help reduce stress and anxiety, which are major risk factors for heart disease.

Some specific chair yoga poses that can benefit heart **health and circulation** include:

- Chair leg raises (improves circulation and strengthens legs)
- Chair arm circles (improves circulation and strengthens arms)
- Chair torso twists (improves circulation and flexibility)
- Chair forward bends (stretches back, shoulders, and hips)
- Chair deep breathing exercises (reduces stress and promotes relaxation)

Chair Yoga Routines

Energizing Morning Chair Yoga

- **Chair Mountain Pose (Upright Seated Pose)**

This is a foundational chair yoga pose that promotes good posture, engages your core, and helps establish a sense of grounding and balance. Here's how to practice it:

1. Sit comfortably in a chair with your feet planted firmly on the ground or a block.
2. Engage your core muscles by drawing your navel towards your spine.
3. Lengthen your spine, imagining a string pulling your head towards the ceiling.
4. Relax your shoulders and keep them down and away from your ears.
5. Place your hands on your thighs or armrests, with your elbows relaxed.

6. Take a few deep breaths, feeling the stability and support of the chair.
7. Gaze forward, keeping your eyes level and soft.

Benefits:

- Improves posture and reduces slouching
- Engages core muscles and promotes stability
- Helps establish balance and grounding
- Relaxes shoulders and reduces tension
- Prepares the body for other chair yoga poses

- **Chair Neck Stretch**

1. Sit comfortably in a chair with your feet planted firmly on the ground or a block.

2. Slowly tilt your head to the right, bringing your ear towards your right shoulder.
3. Keep your chin parallel to the ground and avoid tilting your head forward or backward.
4. Hold the stretch for 30 seconds, breathing deeply and feeling the stretch in your neck and shoulder.
5. Gradually return to the starting position and repeat on the left side.

Tips:

- Keep your shoulders relaxed and down, avoiding scrunching or tensing.
- Breathe deeply and slowly, feeling the stretch deepen with each exhale.
- Don't bounce or force the stretch, as this can cause discomfort or injury.
- Repeat the stretch 2-3 times on each side, as needed.

Benefits:

- Gently stretches the neck and shoulder muscles
- Relaxes tension and reduces stress
- Improves flexibility and range of motion
- Enhances posture and reduces forward head position.

- **Chair Shoulder Rolls**

1. Sit comfortably in a chair with your feet planted firmly on the ground or a block.
2. Roll your shoulders forward and up towards your ears, then back and down, creating a circular motion.
3. Repeat the motion for 30 seconds to 1 minute, breathing deeply and slowly.
4. Focus on relaxing your shoulders and letting go of any tension or stress.

Tips:

- Keep your arms relaxed and let your shoulders do the work.
- Avoid scrunching or tensing your shoulders, as this can create more tension.
- Repeat the rolls several times, as needed, to release tension and improve flexibility.

Benefits:

- Relaxes and loosens the shoulders, reducing tension and stress.
- Improves flexibility and range of motion in the shoulder joint.
- Enhances posture and reduces slouching or hunching.
- Promotes relaxation and reduces muscle fatigue.

- **Chair Chest Expansion**

1. Sit comfortably in a chair with your feet planted firmly on the ground or a block.
2. Place your hands on the armrests or edges of the chair.
3. Take a deep breath in, and as you exhale, gently press your chest forward, stretching your shoulders and chest.
4. Keep your shoulders down and away from your ears, avoiding scrunching or tensing.
5. Hold the expansion for 30 seconds to 1 minute, breathing deeply and slowly.
6. Repeat the expansion several times, as needed, to release tension and improve flexibility.

Tips:

- Keep your spine long and relaxed, avoiding slouching or leaning forward.

- Focus on expanding your chest and shoulders, rather than arching your back.
- Breathe deeply and slowly, feeling the stretch and relaxation spread through your chest and shoulders.

Benefits:

- Opens up the chest and shoulders, promoting flexibility and relaxation.
- Reduces tension and stress in the upper back and shoulders.
- Improves posture and reduces slouching or hunching.
- Enhances breathing and promotes deeper, fuller breaths.

- **Chair Cat-Cow Pose**

1. Sit comfortably in a chair with your feet planted firmly on the ground or a block.
2. Inhale and arch your back, looking up towards the ceiling (like a cat). Keep your shoulders relaxed and down.
3. Exhale and round your back, tucking your chin towards your chest (like a cow). Keep your shoulders relaxed and down.
4. Repeat the sequence several times, moving slowly and smoothly.
5. Continue for 30 seconds to 1 minute, breathing deeply and slowly.

Tips:

- Keep your movements slow and controlled, avoiding jerky or bouncy movements.
- Focus on the gentle arching and rounding of your back, rather than forcing or straining.

- Breathe deeply and slowly, feeling the stretch and relaxation spread through your spine and shoulders.

Benefits:

- Gently warms up the spine and improves flexibility.
- Relaxes and reduces tension in the neck, shoulders, and upper back.
- Promotes relaxation and reduces stress.
- Improves posture and reduces slouching or hunching.

- **Chair Leg Stretch**

1. Sit comfortably in a chair with your feet planted firmly on the ground or a block.

2. Lift one leg out to the side, keeping your foot flexed.
3. Hold the stretch for 30 seconds to 1 minute, breathing deeply and slowly.
4. Slowly lower your leg back down to the starting position.
5. Repeat the stretch on the other side.

Tips:

- Keep your knee straight and your foot flexed.
- Avoid bouncing or forcing the stretch.
- Breathe deeply and slowly, feeling the stretch in your leg and hip.
- Repeat the stretch several times, as needed, to release tension and improve flexibility.

Benefits:

- Stretches the legs, hips, and lower back.

- Relaxes and reduces tension in the legs and hips.
- Improves flexibility and range of motion.
- Enhances circulation and reduces swelling in the legs.

- **Chair Ankle Rotations**

1. Sit comfortably in a chair with your feet planted firmly on the ground or a block.
2. Lift your feet off the ground, keeping your knees straight.
3. Rotate your ankles in a circular motion, first clockwise and then counterclockwise.
4. Repeat the rotation for 30 seconds to 1 minute, breathing deeply and slowly.
5. Slowly lower your feet back down to the starting position.

Tips:

- Keep your knees straight and your feet relaxed.
- Avoid bouncing or forcing the rotation.
- Breathe deeply and slowly, feeling the rotation in your ankles.
- Repeat the rotation several times, as needed, to release tension and improve flexibility.

Benefits:

- Improves ankle mobility and flexibility.
- Relaxes and reduces tension in the feet and ankles.
- Enhances circulation and reduces swelling in the feet and ankles.
- Helps prevent ankle stiffness and injury.

- **Chair Wrist Extensions**

1. Sit comfortably in a chair with your feet planted firmly on the ground or a block.
2. Hold your arms straight out in front of you, with your palms facing down.
3. Slowly tilt your wrists up, keeping your arms straight, and then slowly lower them back down.
4. Repeat the motion for 30 seconds to 1 minute, breathing deeply and slowly.
5. Repeat the sequence several times, as needed, to release tension and improve flexibility.

Tips:

- Keep your arms straight and your shoulders relaxed.
- Avoid bouncing or forcing the motion.
- Breathe deeply and slowly, feeling the stretch in your wrists.

- Repeat the sequence several times, as needed, to release tension and improve flexibility.

Benefits:

- Stretches and mobilizes the wrists and forearms.
- Relaxes and reduces tension in the hands and wrists.
- Improves flexibility and range of motion in the wrists.
- Enhances circulation and reduces swelling in the hands and wrists.

- **Chair Deep Breathing**

1. Sit comfortably in a chair with your feet planted firmly on the ground or a block.

2. Close your eyes and take a slow, deep breath in through your nose, filling your lungs completely.
3. Hold the breath for a few seconds, feeling your body relax and calm.
4. Slowly exhale through your mouth, emptying your lungs completely.
5. Repeat the cycle for several minutes, focusing on your breath and letting go of any thoughts or distractions.

Tips:

- Keep your back straight and your body relaxed.
- Breathe deeply and slowly, feeling your diaphragm expand and contract.
- Avoid shallow or rapid breathing.
- Focus on the sensation of the breath moving in and out of your body.

Benefits:

- Reduces stress and anxiety.

- Promotes relaxation and calmness.
- Improves oxygenation of the body.
- Enhances focus and concentration.
- Supports overall well-being.

Chair Seated Forward Fold

1. Sit comfortably in a chair with your feet planted firmly on the ground or a block.
2. Slowly lean forward, keeping your knees straight, and stretch your arms out in front of you.
3. Lower your forehead towards your hands or knees, keeping your neck relaxed.
4. Hold the stretch for 30 seconds to 1 minute, breathing deeply and slowly.
5. Slowly return to the starting position.

Tips:

- Keep your knees straight and your feet grounded.
- Avoid bouncing or forcing the stretch.
- Breathe deeply and slowly, feeling the stretch in your neck, shoulders, and upper back.
- Repeat the stretch several times, as needed, to release tension and improve flexibility.

Benefits:

- Stretches the neck, shoulders, and upper back.
- Relaxes and reduces tension in the neck and shoulders.
- Improves flexibility and range of motion in the neck and shoulders.
- Enhances circulation and reduces stress.

Afternoon Stress Relief Flow

The morning and afternoon routines are identical, with the same activities and objectives. This consistency is intentional, as it allows for a sense of continuity and routine throughout the day. By repeating the same routine in the morning and afternoon, we can maintain a consistent daily structure and promote a sense of stability and familiarity.

1. **Chair Neck Stretch:** Slowly tilt your head to the right, bringing your ear towards your right shoulder. Hold for 30 seconds and repeat on the left side.

2. **Chair Shoulder Rolls:** Roll your shoulders forward and up towards your ears, then back and down. Repeat for 30 seconds.

3. **Chair Chest Expansion:** Place your hands on the armrests and gently press your chest forward, stretching your shoulders and chest. Hold for 30 seconds.

4. **Chair Cat-Cow Pose:** Arch your back, looking up towards the ceiling (like a cat). Then, round your back, tucking your chin towards your chest (like a cow). Repeat for 30 seconds.

5. **Chair Deep Breathing:** Close your eyes and take slow, deep breaths in through your nose and out through your mouth. Focus on the sensation of the breath. Repeat for 1-2 minutes.

6. **Chair Seated Forward Fold:** Slowly lean forward, stretching your arms out in front of you. Lower your forehead towards your hands or knees, keeping your neck relaxed. Hold for 30 seconds to 1 minute.

7. **Chair Leg Stretch:** Lift one leg out to the side, keeping your foot flexed. Hold for 30 seconds and repeat on the other side.

8. **Chair Ankle Rotations:** Lift your feet off the ground and rotate your ankles in a circular motion, first clockwise and then counterclockwise. Repeat for 30 seconds.

9. **Chair Wrist Extensions:** Hold your arms straight out in front of you and tilt your wrists up and down. Repeat for 30 seconds.

10. **Final Deep Breathing:** Close your eyes and take a few more slow, deep breaths, feeling relaxed and calm.

Evening Relaxation Routine

1. Dim the Lights:

Create a peaceful ambiance by dimming the lights and lighting some calming candles or essential oils.

2. Chair Deep Breathing:

Sit comfortably in a chair and take slow, deep breaths in through your nose and out through your mouth. Focus on the sensation of the breath. Repeat for 5-10 minutes.

3. Neck and Shoulder Release:

Gently roll your shoulders forward and up towards your ears, then back and down. Repeat for 30 seconds. Then, slowly tilt your head to the right, bringing your ear towards your right shoulder. Hold for 30 seconds and repeat on the left side.

4. Chair Leg Stretch:

Lift one leg out to the side, keeping your foot flexed. Hold for 30 seconds and repeat on the other side.

5. Calming Tea or Herbal Infusion:

Enjoy a soothing cup of tea, such as chamomile or lavender, to promote relaxation.

6. Guided Imagery or Meditation:

Listen to a calming guided imagery or meditation recording to quiet your mind and promote relaxation. Repeat for 10-15 minutes.

7. Final Deep Breathing:

Take a few more slow, deep breaths, feeling relaxed and calm.

8. Bedtime Routine:

Gradually transition to your bedtime routine, feeling refreshed and prepared for a restful night's sleep.

Modifying and Adapting Chair Yoga Poses

1. **Modify depth and range:**

For those with limited mobility or flexibility,
reduce the depth and range of motion in
poses.

2. **Use support:**

Utilize chair arms, walls, or blocks for
support and balance in poses.

3. **Shorten holds:**

Reduce the duration of pose holds for those
with fatigue or discomfort.

4. **Choose alternative poses:**

Substitute poses that may be challenging or
uncomfortable with alternative options.

5. Focus on breathing:

Emphasize deep, conscious breathing in poses, especially for those with physical limitations.

6. Listen to your body:

Encourage individuals to honor their body's limitations and rest or modify when needed.

7. Seated or standing options:

Offer both seated and standing options for poses, allowing individuals to choose their preferred position.

8. Assistive devices:

Allow the use of assistive devices like canes, walkers, or wheelchairs to facilitate participation.

9. Gentle transitions:

Encourage gentle, slow transitions between poses to maintain comfort and balance.

10. Encourage self-awareness:

Encourage individuals to tune into their body's needs and adjust poses accordingly.

Using Props for Support and Comfort

1. **Blocks:** Used for support and balance in poses, helping to maintain proper alignment.
2. **Straps:** Assist with deepening stretches or maintaining poses, especially for those with flexibility limitations.
3. **Blankets or Towels:** Provide cushioning and grip for hands and feet in poses.
4. **Pillows or Bolsters:** Support the back, neck, or legs in relaxing poses.
5. **Chair Arms:** Utilize the chair arms for support and balance in poses.
6. **Walls:** Use the wall for support and balance in standing poses or for deepening stretches.
7. **Footrests or Floor Blocks:** Elevate the feet for comfort and support in seated poses.

8. **Eye Pillows or Masks:** Enhance relaxation and reduce visual distractions.
9. **Weighted Blankets:** Provide a calming, grounding sensation for a more relaxing practice.
10. **Heat or Cold Packs:** Relieve tension and discomfort in the muscles and joints.

Progressing Towards Advanced Variations

1. Master the basics:

Ensure a strong foundation in fundamental chair yoga poses and breathing techniques.

2. Build strength and flexibility:

Gradually increase your strength and flexibility through regular practice and modification of poses.

3. Introduce gentle flows:

Progress from static poses to gentle flows, linking movements with breath.

4. Advance to deeper stretches:

Gradually deepen stretches, using props and modifications as needed.

5. Incorporate balance and coordination:

Introduce balance poses and movements that challenge coordination.

6. Explore dynamic movements:

Progress to dynamic movements, like chair sun salutations and flowing sequences.

7. Refine alignment and technique:

Focus on precise alignment, engagement of core muscles, and efficient breathing.

8. Incorporate props and weights:

Utilize props and weights to enhance strength, balance, and flexibility.

9. Practice advanced breathing techniques:

Explore advanced pranayama practices, like alternate nostril breathing and kapalabhati.

10. Embrace mindfulness and meditation:

Deepen your practice with mindfulness and meditation techniques, cultivating inner awareness and calm.

Remember to:

- Listen to your body and modify or rest when needed.
- Practice regularly to build strength, flexibility, and endurance.
- Seek guidance from experienced instructors or online resources.
- Honor your limitations and progress at your own pace.

Addressing Women's Concerns and Questions

Exploring Health and Fitness Myths

- **You can target your fat burn:** You can't control what part of your body burns the most fat.
- **Lifting heavy weights bulks up women:** Lifting weights tones and shapes your body.
- **Crunches are the best moves for your core:** Increase your cardio workouts and add resistance training that targets the entire core.
- **Exercise can erase a bad diet:** Diet and nutrition play a larger role than exercise in weight management and cancer prevention.
- **When you stop strength training, muscle turns to fat:** When you stop

strength training, you lose muscle mass and your metabolism slows down.

- **You need to spend hours in the gym:** You can get all the benefits of exercise whether you're at the gym or at home.
- **Stretch before exercising:** It's more effective to stretch after you exercise when your muscles and joints are warm.
- **More sweat equals a better workout:** Sweat occurs in an effort to regulate your body's core temperature.
- **If you don't feel sore right away after an exercise, it isn't a good one:** Some workouts cause a burning feeling right after you finish them, while others can take several days before delayed onset muscle soreness (DOMS) sets in.
- **You can eat as much junk food as you want as long as you exercise:**

Consuming a lot of junk food will have negative consequences for your body.

Solutions to some Common challenges

Challenge: Limited mobility or flexibility
Solution: Modify poses, use props, and focus on breathing and relaxation techniques.

Challenge: Back pain or discomfort
Solution: Strengthen core muscles, engage in gentle twists and stretches, and use supportive props.

Challenge: Balance or coordination issues
Solution: Use chair arms or walls for support, practice balance poses with feet hip-width apart, and focus on slow, controlled movements.

Challenge: Fatigue or low energy

Solution: Practice gentle, restorative poses, incorporate deep breathing and relaxation techniques, and take regular breaks.

Challenge: Limited range of motion in shoulders or hips
Solution: Use props to support and deepen stretches, practice gentle rotations and mobilizations, and focus on building strength and flexibility.

Challenge: Difficulty quieting the mind or finding focus
Solution: Practice mindfulness meditation, use guided imagery or visualization techniques, and focus on the breath or physical sensations in the body.

Additional Resources for Learning

Congratulations on completing this chair yoga journey! To continue your practice beyond this book, consider the following:

1. Explore online resources:

Websites like YouTube, Yoga International, and DoYouYoga offer a vast array of chair yoga classes and tutorials.

2. Invest in yoga props:

Enhance your practice with blocks, straps, blankets, and bolsters to deepen stretches and maintain proper alignment.

3. Join a local yoga studio or class:

Connect with experienced instructors and like-minded individuals to diversify your practice and gain new insights.

4. Attend workshops and retreats:

Deepen your understanding of yoga philosophy, anatomy, and teaching techniques.

5. Practice regularly:

Aim for consistency, even if it's just a few minutes each day, to cultivate a lasting habit and experience the full benefits of yoga.

6. Modify and adapt:

Continue to listen to your body and modify poses as needed, exploring new variations and props to keep your practice fresh and engaging.

7. Share your practice:

Introduce friends and family to chair yoga, and consider teaching or assisting others to deepen your understanding and connection with the practice.

8. Embrace mindfulness and meditation:

Incorporate these practices into your daily routine to enhance your overall well-being and complement your physical yoga practice.

9. Seek guidance and mentorship:

Connect with experienced yoga instructors or mentors for personalized guidance and support.

10.   Keep exploring and learning:

Stay curious and open to new techniques, philosophies, and styles to continue growing and evolving in your yoga journey.

Conclusion

Reflecting on Your Chair Yoga Journey

Congratulations on completing your chair yoga journey! Take a moment to reflect on your experience:

- What drew you to chair yoga, and what were your initial expectations?

- How has your physical practice evolved over time? Have you noticed improvements in flexibility, strength, or balance?

- What mental and emotional benefits have you experienced through chair yoga, such as reduced stress or increased calmness?

- How has chair yoga impacted your daily life, including your relationships, work, or overall well-being?

- What challenges did you face, and how did you overcome them?

- What are your favorite chair yoga poses or sequences, and why?

- How has your understanding of yoga philosophy and breathing techniques deepened?

- What goals or intentions do you have for continuing your chair yoga practice?

- How has chair yoga influenced your self-awareness, self-acceptance, and self-compassion?

- What gratitude do you have for your body, mind, and spirit, and for the chair yoga practice itself?

Final Thoughts and Encouragement

- Be gentle and compassionate with yourself.

- Celebrate your small victories and accomplishments.

- Embrace your journey, and don't compare yourself to others.

- Remember, yoga is not just a physical practice, but a mental and spiritual one too.

- Take your time, and don't rush your practice.

- Breathe, relax, and enjoy the journey!

- Keep exploring, learning, and growing.

- Share your practice with others, and inspire them to start their own journey.

- Most importantly, have fun and be kind to yourself!

Appendix

Some Common Yoga terms:

1. **Abhyasa:** the act of practicing
2. **Acharya:** teacher
3. **Adwaita:** a philosophy that says there is no duality, only a singular state of consciousness
4. **Agni:** fire
5. **Ahimsa:** non-violence, non-injury, one of the yamas of ashtanga yoga
6. **Ajna chakra:** energy center located behind the forehead, also called psychic center, one of the seven energy centers
7. **Akasha:** ether, space
8. **Anahata chakra:** energy center located in the heart region, also called pranic centre, fourth of the seven energy centers
9. **Ananda:** bliss, ecstasy

10. **Asana:** yoga position or yoga pose, also called yogasana, a balanced position for smooth energy flow in specific areas of the body and mind

11. **Ashrama:** residential place of people living together in yogic tradition

12. **Ashtanga yoga:** the eight fold path of yoga as outlined by Patanjali: yama, niyama, asana, pranayama, pratyahara, dharana, dhyana, samadhi

13. **Ashwini mudra:** practice of contracting the anal sphincter

14. **Atman:** soul

15. **Aum:** see Om

Author's Note

To all the wonderful readers who have journeyed through the pages of this book, I extend my heartfelt gratitude and warmest wishes. Your decision to explore the transformative practice of chair yoga speaks volumes about your commitment to self-care, well-being, and personal growth.

As you hold this book in your hands, may you feel a sense of empowerment and possibility, knowing that you have the tools and wisdom within you to cultivate greater balance, comfort, and joy in your life. May the practices and insights shared here serve as a guiding light on your path to health, happiness, and wholeness.

Remember, you are the author of your own story, and each moment is an opportunity to create the life you desire. Whether you're embarking on a new journey of self-discovery or deepening your existing practice, may you find inspiration, support, and encouragement within these pages.

As you integrate the teachings of chair yoga into your daily life, may you experience a profound sense of connection—to yourself, to others, and to the world around you. May you embrace the beauty of each breath, each movement, and each moment, knowing that you are deserving of love, kindness, and compassion.

Thank you for choosing to embark on this journey with me. May your heart be filled with gratitude, your spirit be lifted with joy, and your life be enriched with abundance.

With warmest regards and deepest appreciation,

Christoph Hermann

GET ACCESS TO MY OTHER BOOKS

BY SCANNING THE QR CODE ABOVE

www.ingramcontent.com/pod-product-compliance
Lightning Source LLC
Chambersburg PA
CBHW051614250726
48653CB00004BA/1511